TRADITIONAL CHINESE MEDICINE

A Comprehensive Guide To (TCM) Diagnostic Methods, Treatment Modalities, Common Conditions, Integrative Approaches, Modern Applications And Challenges

WILFREDO CARSON

INTRODUCTION

Traditional Chinese Medicine (TCM) is a rich and ancient method of healing that has evolved over millennia. Its origins run deep in Chinese history and culture, and it has a tremendous impact on people's health and well-being.

This complete system takes a holistic approach, incorporating therapies like acupuncture, herbal medicine, massage, and food therapy. Understanding TCM's origins, philosophy, and historical development is essential for grasping its complexities and the principles that underlie its methods.

Background of Traditional Chinese Medicine

Traditional Chinese Medicine has thousands of years of history and is firmly rooted in Chinese philosophy, culture, and spirituality.

TCM is based on the ancient Chinese belief in the balance of Yin and Yang, the flow of Qi (vital energy), and the connectivity of the body, mind, and spirit. Early practitioners studied the natural environment to better grasp the principles that regulate health and disease.

The Huangdi Neijing, or Yellow Emperor's Inner Canon, is a foundational document in TCM that provides insights into the medical system's holistic approach. It dates back to the third century BCE.

The use of herbal treatments, acupuncture, and other medicinal techniques became commonplace, demonstrating the significant influence of Chinese cosmology on healthcare.

Philosophy and Principles of Traditional Chinese Medicine

TCM philosophy revolves around the concept of Qi, the vital energy that runs through the body's meridians, influencing health and sustaining equilibrium.

The concept covers the interaction of Yin and Yang, opposing but complementary forces that exist in a dynamic balance. TCM practitioners see the body as a microcosm of the broader cosmos, and imbalances in Yin and Yang or disturbances in Qi flow are said to cause illness.

The Five Elements theory, another TCM pillar, divides the body's functions and structures into Wood, Fire, Earth, Metal, and Water elements, reflecting their interrelationships.

 In TCM, diagnosis entails recognizing patterns of disharmony while taking into account aspects such as Qi quality, Yin and Yang state, and Five Elements balance. Acupuncture, herbal therapy, and other techniques customized to the individual's particular constitution are used as treatment strategies to restore balance and harmony.

Historical Development and Evolution.TCM has evolved dynamically, influenced by numerous dynasties, philosophical upheavals, and cultural changes throughout Chinese history.

The combination of Taoist and Confucian concepts, combined with the exchange of medical knowledge along the Silk Road, strengthened TCM's theoretical roots. During the Tang and Song dynasties, medical treatises and encyclopedias were created to consolidate and systematize TCM knowledge. Notable physicians, such as Zhang Zhongjing and Li Shizhen, made substantial contributions to herbal therapy by prescribing formulations that are being used today.

Further improvements occurred in the twentieth century, as TCM was modernized and integrated into China's healthcare system. Efforts were made to standardize diagnostic criteria, improve education, and conduct scientific research into TCM modalities.

TCM is already widely recognized around the world, with a growing interest in its holistic approach and possible complementarity to Western treatment.

Finally, Traditional Chinese Medicine is a profound and holistic approach to healthcare that is based on ancient ideas and has been modified by millennia of cultural and historical events.

Understanding its history, philosophy, and evolution is critical to appreciating the breadth and complexity of this traditional therapeutic practice. TCM continues to play an important role in modern healthcare by providing a unique viewpoint on the interdependence of the body, mind, and spirit.

CHAPTER 1
FUNDAMENTALS OF TRADITIONAL CHINESE MEDICINE

Yin-Yang Theory:

The Yin and Yang theory is a foundation of Traditional Chinese Medicine (TCM), providing a comprehensive view of the nature of existence and health. This ancient Chinese philosophical notion is founded on the premise that the world is made up of dualistic energies, represented by Yin and Yang. Yin symbolizes the feminine, dark, and passive features, and Yang represents the masculine, brilliant, and energetic attributes. TCM views health as a dynamic balance between these conflicting forces. Balance and harmony between Yin and Yang are essential for overall well-being.

<u>Balance and harmony:</u>

The essence of the Yin and Yang theory is to achieve balance and harmony inside the body. In Traditional Chinese Medicine, the body is viewed as a microcosm of the cosmos, and any imbalance between Yin and Yang can cause discord and illness. Practitioners work to understand each individual's unique constitution and determine imbalances by examining symptoms, pulse, and tongue features. The goal is to restore homeostasis via acupuncture, herbal medicine, and lifestyle changes.

<u>Interconnected Opposites:</u>

The interconnectivity of Yin and Yang stresses their mutual dependency and ongoing interaction. This concept recognizes that one cannot exist without the other and that their relationship is dynamic rather than static. For example, excess Yin can turn into Yang and vice versa. TCM practitioners use this information to develop therapies that address the underlying cause of imbalances and restore the body's balanced energy flow.

Five Elements Theory:

The Five Elements theory, commonly known as Wu Xing, is another key idea in Traditional Chinese Medicine that provides a framework for understanding the relationships and interactions between the natural world and the human body.

Wood, Fire, Earth, Metal, and Water:

The Five Elements (Wood, Fire, Earth, Metal, and Water) represent various aspects of nature and their associated traits. Each element corresponds to a specific physical organ, season, color, flavor, and emotion.

For example, Wood is associated with the liver, spring, green, sour flavor, and the feeling of fury. Understanding these correspondences enables TCM practitioners to examine symptoms and discover imbalances associated with specific elements, hence directing the development of tailored treatment programs.

Relationship with body organs and functions:

The Five Elements theory's influence extends to the organs and their activities in the human body. Each element oversees a specific organ system, regulating both physiological and pathological processes. This interconnectivity underscores TCM's holistic approach, which considers the balance of the entire system to sustain health.

For example, imbalances in the Wood element may impact the liver and gallbladder, resulting in symptoms such as digestive problems or mental distress.

Qi (or vital energy) and blood:

Qi, often known as vital energy, is a central concept in TCM that governs the dynamic activities of the human body. Qi flows through a network of channels and meridians, promoting balance and overall health. Understanding the circulation and balance of Qi is critical for TCM practitioners who diagnose and treat a variety of health issues.

Circulation and Balance:

In TCM, the smooth circulation of Qi is critical for good health. Any interruption or stagnation of Qi can cause discord and sickness.

To regulate Qi flow and restore balance, practitioners employ acupuncture, herbal medicine, and other techniques.

The idea of Qi circulation encompasses both mental and emotional aspects, underlining TCM's holistic character.

<u>Channels and meridians:</u>

In TCM, channels and meridians reflect the pathways via which Qi and Blood circulate, linking different areas of the body.

These pathways comprise a complex network that connects organs, tissues, and physiological activities. TCM practitioners employ acupuncture to stimulate specific spots along these channels, supporting a smooth flow of Qi and correcting imbalances.

The concept of channels and meridians is central to TCM diagnosis and treatment procedures, allowing practitioners to recognize patterns of imbalance and customize interventions accordingly.

the principles of Traditional Chinese Medicine, which include the Yin and Yang theory, the Five Elements theory, and the notions of Qi and blood circulation through channels and meridians, provide a comprehensive and interrelated knowledge of health and well-being. TCM's holistic approach focuses on the dynamic balance of opposing forces, the harmonious interplay of natural elements, and the vital energy that supports life. This ancient system remains a useful and growing foundation for promoting health, preventing illness, and treating a variety of ailments.

pg. 15

CHAPTER 2
DIAGNOSTIC METHODS IN TCM

Diagnostic methods in Traditional Chinese Medicine (TCM) are critical for identifying underlying imbalances in the body and developing effective treatment regimens. These treatments are profoundly entrenched in TCM's holistic approach, which considers the body, mind, and spirit to be interrelated. TCM practitioners' primary diagnostic tools include observation, hearing and smelling, inquiry, and pulse diagnosis.

Observation, as described by the ancient Chinese medical scholar Wang, is an important diagnostic approach in TCM. Facial diagnosis, a type of observation, is examining facial features for symptoms of interior imbalances. Practitioners evaluate the color, texture, and expression of the face to gather information on the state of numerous organs and systems. Tongue diagnosis, another aspect of observation, involves a thorough study of the tongue's color, coating, shape, and moisture. In TCM, the tongue is viewed as a mirror reflecting the internal state of organs, assisting in the detection of imbalances and guiding treatment techniques.

Listening and smelling, sometimes known as "Wen," are diagnostic approaches that rely on detecting small indications from patients. Sound and odor diagnostics entails listening intently to the patient's voice and smelling any distinctive odors emerging from the body. Changes in the quality, tone, or pitch of the voice, as well as peculiar scents, are thought to indicate imbalances in specific organs or meridians.

These procedures provide useful information regarding the patient's internal state and contribute to a more complete diagnostic picture.

Inquiry, another important diagnostic procedure in TCM, entails a comprehensive examination of the patient's history and symptoms. The concepts of "Wen," which emphasize the significance of communication between the practitioner and the patient, led to this procedure. The patient's history, which includes characteristics like as lifestyle, diet, and emotional well-being, assists the practitioner in understanding the individual's constitution and probable contributing causes to the current condition. Symptom evaluation entails a thorough investigation into the nature, duration, and intensity of symptoms, allowing the practitioner to find trends and develop a tailored treatment strategy.

Pulse diagnosis is a distinguishing element of TCM, and mastery is regarded as a sign of a skilled practitioner. Identifying imbalances using pulse diagnostics entails palpating radial pulses at several locations, each of which corresponds to a distinct organ or meridians. Practitioners examine the depth, rate, strength, and quality of the pulse to determine the status of Qi and Blood in the body. The interpretation of pulse characteristics improves the diagnostic procedure by providing insights into the nature of imbalances and directing the selection of acupuncture points or herbal medicines.

Finally, Traditional Chinese Medicine's diagnostic methods reflect a comprehensive and patient-centered approach to healthcare. Observation, hearing and smelling, inquiry, and pulse diagnosis all contribute to a complete framework for comprehending the complex interactions between the body's numerous systems. These methods not only help to discover current imbalances, but they also allow for a better knowledge of an individual's constitution and the elements that contribute to their health. The combination of these diagnostic methods demonstrates TCM's holistic concept, which views the body as an integrated system impacted by the dynamic interaction of Qi, Blood, and the fundamental principles of Yin and Yang.

CHAPTER 3
TCM TREATMENT MODALITIES

Traditional Chinese Medicine (TCM) comprises a wide range of treatment approaches, each with a solid foundation in ancient Chinese philosophy and medical concepts. Among these techniques, acupuncture stands out as a cornerstone, representing the delicate balance of energy throughout the body. Acupuncture involves inserting thin needles into particular locations along the body's meridians, which are pathways that carry vital energy, or Qi.

The meridians constitute a complex network, with acupoints chosen based on the patient's ailment. This method seeks to control the flow of Qi, so restoring balance and boosting general health. A precise understanding of meridians and acupoints is critical to the efficiency of acupuncture.

Meridians act as routes for the passage of Qi, linking various organs and tissues.

The concept of meridians is fundamental to Chinese medicine's understanding of the body's energy system. There are twelve main meridians, each connected with a certain organ and representing a different component of the body's operations. Acupoints, or precise points along these meridians, are carefully selected depending on the patient's symptoms and the underlying imbalance in their Qi. The selection of acupoints necessitates a thorough grasp of the body's interconnection as well as the Yin and Yang principles, which control the body's opposing but complementary forces.

The techniques and equipment used in acupuncture demonstrate the intricacy and sophistication of this TCM treatment. Acupuncture needles, usually made of stainless steel, are inserted at certain angles and depths to promote the flow of Qi.

To increase the therapeutic results, practitioners may employ a variety of techniques, including physical manipulation and electrical stimulation. The utilization of acupuncture tools, such as plum blossom needles or moxibustion, expands the therapy options. Plum blossom needles require touching the skin's surface with a little device to stimulate blood circulation and Qi flow. In contrast, moxibustion is the practice of burning dried mugwort at acupoints to generate heat and encourage energy flow. These approaches highlight the vast range of treatments used in acupuncture, showing its applicability to a variety of health issues.

Herbal medicine is another important aspect of TCM, drawing on a diverse pharmacopeia of plants, minerals, and animal products. Classic formulae are the foundation of herbal medicines, combining many substances to address complicated health issues. These formulae, established over millennia, embody TCM's holistic principles and strive to balance the body's inherent dynamics. Single herbs and mixtures offer a complex approach to treatment, with each plant having distinct qualities and activities. The combination of herbs in a mix boosts their medicinal effects while reducing potential negative effects.

Herb selection and combination are governed by TCM diagnosis concepts, which identify patterns of disharmony based on the patient's constitution and symptoms.

Classic formulae, such as the well-known "Si Jun Zi Tang" for tonifying Qi, demonstrate the methodical approach to herbal treatment. Si Jun Zi Tang includes four herbs, each of which adds to the formula's overall effectiveness. Ginseng, a crucial element, tonifies Qi, while the other herbs support its effect by addressing various parts of the patient's condition. This holistic approach distinguishes TCM herbal treatment from traditional pharmaceutical techniques by stressing individualized and balanced formulations based on the individual's unique constitution.

Cupping therapy, a unique TCM method, includes the use of suction cups on the skin's surface. This technique creates a vacuum, which improves blood circulation and Qi flow. Glass, bamboo, and plastic are all options for cup materials. The therapy is intended to alleviate stagnation, disperse cold or dampness, and stimulate the body's natural healing processes. Cupping is frequently used to relieve musculoskeletal pain, increase detoxification, and improve general health. The characteristic round marks left on the skin during cupping, known as "cupping marks" or "sha," are regarded as therapeutic indicators that indicate the release of pathogenic elements.

Tui Na, often known as Chinese massage, is a hands-on treatment practice within TCM. This modality uses a variety of manual techniques, such as kneading, pushing, and stretching, to manipulate the body's soft tissues and encourage energy flow.

Tui Na and acupuncture have similar theoretical roots, with a focus on the meridian system and Qi regulation. Practitioners use particular procedures tailored to the patient's condition, addressing both local and systemic imbalances. Tui Na is used to treat a variety of maladies, including musculoskeletal difficulties, digestive problems, and stress-related illnesses. Its efficacy is based on its ability to balance the body's energy and address the underlying causes of illness.

Qi Gong and Tai Chi are mind-body techniques with roots in Chinese philosophy and martial arts traditions. These practices include intentional movements, breath control, and meditation to cultivate Qi, boost vitality, and promote overall well-being. Qi Gong includes a wide range of activities, such as fixed postures, dynamic motions, and meditation.

The emphasis is on synchronizing breath and movement to balance the Yin and Yang forces in the body. Tai Chi, a martial art style based on Qi Gong principles, stresses gentle, flowing movements that involve the full body. Both Qi Gong and Tai Chi promote physical and mental health by lowering stress, improving balance, and increasing total energy flow.

The therapeutic benefits of Qi Gong and Tai Chi go beyond physical health to include mental and emotional well-being.

These practices are recognized as helpful stress management techniques that promote relaxation and mental clarity. Qi cultivation through mindful movement and breathwork promotes a deep connection between the body and mind, which aids emotional balance and resilience. Qi Gong and Tai Chi have been shown in studies to improve a variety of health issues, including cardiovascular health, chronic pain, and mental health concerns. The incorporation of these mind-body activities within TCM represents a holistic approach to well-being that recognizes the interdependence of the physical, mental, and emotional elements of health.

To summarize, TCM therapeutic techniques comprise a diverse range of approaches, each profoundly based on ancient wisdom and philosophies. Acupuncture, which focuses on meridians and acupoints, uses a variety of procedures and tools to regulate Qi and restore balance. Herbal medicine, using old formulae and specific herbs, provides a tailored and holistic approach to dealing with the intricacies of health disorders. Cupping therapy, Tui Na, and mind-body therapies such as Qi Gong and Tai Chi all add to the rich tapestry of TCM, improving total well-being through focused interventions and the cultivation of harmonious energy flow. These modalities, with their rich history and ongoing study, continue to play an important part in the global landscape of complementary and alternative medicine.

CHAPTER 4
COMMON TCM CONDITIONS AND TREATMENTS

Traditional Chinese Medicine (TCM) addresses digestive issues holistically, stressing Qi balance and internal organ harmony. Acupuncture and herbal therapies are important in resolving digestive disorders within this context. Acupuncture, which involves inserting small needles into specific sites on the body, aims to reestablish the smooth flow of Qi, relieving symptoms such as bloating, indigestion, and irregular bowel movements.

TCM herbal formulae are also used to rebalance the digestive system by correcting underlying imbalances, such as excess or deficiency in specific organs.

Common herbs such as ginger, peppermint, and licorice are used to calm the digestive system and regulate functions.

The combination of acupuncture and herbal therapies illustrates the holistic TCM approach to digestive issues, which promotes general health by restoring the body's natural balance.

TCM Treatments for Asthma and Respiratory Infections

TCM provides novel views and effective treatments for respiratory diseases, including chronic difficulties such as asthma and acute respiratory infections. In TCM, respiratory health is directly linked to the Lung organ system, which regulates Qi and circulates vital energy. Acupuncture is widely used to stimulate specific spots on the lungs, improving Qi flow and treating underlying imbalances that contribute to respiratory diseases.

Herbal treatments like ma huang (Ephedra sinica) and xing ren (Prunus armeniaca) are used to treat wheezing and coughing.

TCM stresses customized treatment, acknowledging that everyone's constitution and underlying patterns are unique.

This technique attempts to strengthen the respiratory system for long-term health and recurrence prevention, as well as to alleviate current symptoms.

<u>Musculoskeletal Disorders: Pain Management with Acupuncture and Tui Na</u>

Musculoskeletal problems, which are characterized by pain and dysfunction in the muscles, joints, and bones, are efficiently treated in TCM with acupuncture and Tui Na massage.

Acupuncture focuses on specific meridians connected with the problematic areas, encouraging the flow of Qi and blood to relieve pain and inflammation.

The stimulation of acupuncture sites causes the release of endorphins, the body's natural painkillers, which provide relief and restore equilibrium. Tui Na, a type of Chinese therapeutic massage, enhances acupuncture by relieving muscle tension, increasing circulation, and aiding the elimination of meridian blockages. This dual approach not only alleviates pain but also tackles the underlying causes of musculoskeletal diseases, such as Qi and blood stagnation.

TCM's holistic concept ensures that treatments take into account the interconnectivity of many bodily systems to enhance general well-being.

Emotional and mental health: depression, anxiety, and stress management.

Traditional Chinese Medicine acknowledges the close relationship between the body and mind, viewing emotional and mental health as essential components of general well-being. TCM sees emotions as representations of Qi flow and emphasizes the necessity of maintaining a harmonic balance to avoid imbalances that can lead to conditions like depression, anxiety, and tension.

Acupuncture regulates the flow of Qi through specific sites related to emotional well-being, encouraging relaxation and alleviating symptoms connected with mental health issues.

 Herbal formulations, which frequently include adaptogenic herbs such as ginseng and Schisandra, are prescribed to help the nervous system and restore equilibrium. Lifestyle and nutritional recommendations are also important components of TCM interventions for emotional and mental health, emphasizing the value of a balanced and nourishing lifestyle to develop emotional resilience.

Women's Health: Traditional Chinese Medicine in Gynecology and Obstetrics

TCM has a long history of treating women's health issues and understanding the female body's distinct physiological and hormonal characteristics. TCM is used in gynecology and obstetrics to regulate the menstrual cycle, promote fertility, and treat a variety of reproductive disorders. Acupuncture is used to regulate hormone levels, relieve menstruation pain, and improve blood circulation in the reproductive organs.

Herbal formulas suited to particular patterns of imbalance are frequently used to treat illnesses such as irregular menstruation, polycystic ovarian syndrome (PCOS), and endometriosis. TCM also helps women throughout pregnancy by treating typical symptoms including nausea, tiredness, and back pain.

TCM's holistic approach to women's health acknowledges the interplay of physical, emotional, and energetic elements, resulting in a comprehensive framework for optimizing reproductive health.

<u>Fertility and Pregnancy Support</u>

TCM fertility and pregnancy support go beyond traditional biomedical techniques, stressing the body's natural balance as the key to successful conception and a healthy pregnancy. Acupuncture is commonly used to control the menstrual cycle, improve ovarian function, and increase uterine blood flow. Specific acupuncture points are used to treat reproductive issues such as polycystic ovarian syndrome (PCOS) and unexplained infertility. Herbal compositions containing fertility-enhancing herbs like dong quai and shu di huang are used to treat underlying imbalances and nourish the reproductive system. During pregnancy, TCM focuses on the health of both the mother and the developing fetus. Acupuncture can help with common pregnant symptoms like morning sickness and back pain, whereas herbal treatments are tailored to each trimester's specific needs. TCM's holistic approach to conception and pregnancy support acknowledges the complex interplay of physiological, emotional, and energetic aspects, resulting in a tailored and comprehensive approach to reproductive health.

CHAPTER 5
INTEGRATIVE APPROACHES AND MODERN APPLICATIONS

Traditional Chinese Medicine (TCM) has a rich history dating back thousands of years and has grown into a comprehensive healthcare system. In recent years, there has been an increased interest in merging TCM with Western medicine, recognizing the potential benefits of mixing ancient wisdom with modern scientific methodologies.

This integrative approach seeks to deliver more comprehensive and patient-centered care while recognizing the qualities of both systems.

5.1 Integrating TCM and Western Medicine:

The merger of TCM and Western medicine marks a paradigm shift in healthcare, encouraging collaboration between two historically separate medical systems.

This strategy recognizes that each system has distinct strengths and weaknesses, and it seeks to leverage their synergies for the benefit of patient health.

Collaborative healthcare models have arisen as a key component of this integration, in which practitioners from both disciplines collaborate to develop comprehensive treatment programs.

5.1. 1 Models of Collaborative Healthcare:

Collaborative healthcare models that combine TCM and Western medicine stress interdisciplinary communication and cooperation.

In these models, practitioners from both sides contribute their expertise, resulting in a more comprehensive picture of the patient's health. This partnership extends beyond individual patient cases to include research projects, teaching activities, and the creation of standardized practices.

The idea is to combine the assets of each system to address complicated health concerns and improve overall patient outcomes.

5.2 Research and Evidence-Based Practice:

The value of research and evidence-based approaches in the integration of TCM and Western medicine cannot be understated. Scientific research on TCM efficacy has been a key area for establishing legitimacy and closing the gap between traditional knowledge and modern medical norms.

TCM therapies are evaluated using rigorous research procedures to ensure their safety, efficacy, and mechanisms of action, laying the groundwork for successful integration.

5.2.1 Scientific Research on TCM Efficacy:

Numerous scientific researches has looked into the efficacy of TCM interventions and their effects on various health issues.

From acupuncture and herbal medicine to qigong and food therapy, researchers have used randomized controlled trials and systematic reviews to evaluate the efficacy of TCM treatments. This research adds to the expanding body of evidence supporting the integration of TCM into mainstream healthcare, assisting in clinical decision-making and improving patient outcomes.

5.3 TCM and Preventive Medicine:

The preventative side of healthcare is gaining popularity, and TCM provides a unique perspective on overall well-being and illness prevention. Rather than focusing primarily on treating existing ailments, TCM emphasizes the necessity of preserving internal balance and harmony to avoid disease formation.

This preventative strategy is consistent with the rising acknowledgment of the importance of lifestyle and wellness behaviors in promoting overall health.

5.3.1 Holistic Health and Disease Prevention:

In Traditional Chinese Medicine, holistic wellness refers to a wide range of aspects such as physical, mental, and emotional health.

Acupuncture, herbal medicine, and food therapy are utilized not only to treat specific health conditions but also to promote general bodily balance.

TCM attempts to prevent disease by taking into account the interconnection of many body systems. This preventative focus is consistent with modern healthcare methods, which shift the emphasis from reactive treatment to proactive health management.

the merger of Traditional Chinese Medicine and Western Medicine represents a potential frontier in healthcare. Collaborative models, underpinned by rigorous research and evidence-based practices, pave the way for a more holistic and patient-centered approach to therapy. The preventative components of TCM contribute to the changing landscape of healthcare by highlighting the relevance of overall well-being in illness prevention. As these integrative techniques gain traction, they have the potential to form a more inclusive and effective healthcare system that incorporates the best of both traditional and modern medical paradigms.

CHAPTER 6
FUTURE TRENDS AND CHALLENGES

Advancements in TCM scientific: The field of Traditional Chinese Medicine (TCM) is entering a revolutionary phase, with significant scientific advances. One important feature is the unique research of treatment techniques within TCM. Modern scientific procedures, such as molecular and cellular approaches, are being used in TCM research to shed light on the underlying mechanisms of traditional treatments. Researchers are investigating the pharmacological properties of TCM herbs and formulations, discovering active components, and determining their specific physiological effects. This combination of ancient wisdom and modern scientific rigor not only strengthens TCM's credibility but also opens the door to novel treatments. Furthermore, advances in genomics and personalized medicine are influencing TCM research, enabling for more targeted and effective application of traditional medicines. The use of cutting-edge technologies in TCM research confirms traditional techniques while also establishing TCM as a dynamic and expanding field capable of tackling modern healthcare concerns.

Innovations in Treatment Modalities: In TCM's ever-changing landscape, treatment modalities are playing an increasingly important role in molding the future of traditional therapeutic techniques. Traditional Chinese Medicine has long been connected with acupuncture, herbal medicines, and holistic health approaches. However, recent discoveries are broadening the therapeutic options.

Biomedical technology is being used to improve acupuncture treatments, resulting in a more precise and personalized therapeutic experience. Furthermore, TCM is becoming more widely used in conjunction with other complementary and alternative medical techniques. Collaborations between TCM practitioners and Western medical experts are promoting a more holistic approach to patient treatment, leveraging the strengths of both systems. Furthermore, there is a growing interest in investigating the possibilities of TCM in preventative medicine, with an emphasis on lifestyle changes and wellness programs. These advancements not only improve the efficacy of TCM but also contribute to its acceptance in the larger healthcare setting.

Globalization of Traditional Chinese Medicine: The globalization of Traditional Chinese Medicine is a significant movement that has far-reaching consequences for both healthcare practices and cultural interchange. TCM, which has strong roots in Chinese philosophy and customs, is expanding beyond geographical bounds. TCM methods are spreading over the world as more people recognize their holistic approach and possible therapeutic advantages. Beyond China, TCM is gaining popularity in other nations, resulting in the establishment of TCM clinics and academic institutions worldwide.

This globalization is not limited to the spread of treatment techniques; it also includes the adoption of TCM principles into conventional healthcare systems. Collaboration between Chinese and non-Chinese practitioners promotes cross-cultural knowledge exchange, enriching global understanding of healthcare practices. The globalization of TCM symbolizes a harmonic combination of many medical traditions, with the potential to provide a more complete and inclusive approach to healthcare on a global scale.

TCM Practices Around the World: As TCM becomes more globalized, one exciting feature is the adaptation and integration of TCM practices from around the world. Various countries and cultures are implementing TCM concepts into their healthcare systems, frequently combining traditional techniques with conventional medicine. Acupuncture, for example, has become widely accepted as a therapeutic method for a variety of illnesses in Western countries. TCM herbal medicines are also being investigated and used in treatment methods in many medical contexts. This incorporation of TCM procedures into other cultural contexts demonstrates not just the universal appeal of its holistic philosophy, but also the adaptability of traditional healing approaches. However, problems such as standardizing TCM techniques and guaranteeing practitioner competence across many cultural and regulatory contexts must be addressed to promote TCM's harmonic integration into global healthcare practices.

hurdles and Ethical Considerations: Despite potential advances in TCM research and globalization, the field has hurdles and ethical concerns. TCM product consistency and quality control are a substantial issue.

The heterogeneity in herbal formulation composition, as well as the lack of regulated production techniques, make it difficult to ensure the safety and efficacy of TCM treatments. Ethical concerns often arise around the conservation of endangered plant and animal species found in traditional preparations. Another problem is to bridge the gap between TCM's holistic concept and modern medicine's reductionist approach. Integrating TCM into mainstream healthcare necessitates overcoming skepticism and building mutual understanding between TCM practitioners and Western medical experts. Furthermore, concerns concerning the training and regulation of TCM practitioners, particularly in countries where TCM is not deeply based on tradition, require careful examination.

Addressing these problems is critical for the long-term development and ethical practice of TCM on a worldwide basis.

CONCLUSION

The future of Traditional Chinese Medicine (TCM) is defined by a dynamic interaction of scientific advances, innovative treatment methods, globalization, and navigating associated obstacles and ethical considerations. Integrating modern scientific approaches into TCM research increases the legitimacy and applicability of traditional practices. Innovations in therapeutic methods increase TCM's breadth, stimulating collaborations with other medical traditions and contributing to a more holistic approach to patient care. The globalization of TCM demonstrates a harmonious synthesis of many cultural viewpoints on healthcare, expanding worldwide awareness of ancient healing techniques. However, issues with standardization, quality control, and ethical considerations highlight the importance of taking a thorough and thoughtful approach to integrating TCM into mainstream healthcare systems. As TCM evolves and adapts to modern healthcare needs, its ability to provide a holistic and inclusive approach to wellness on a worldwide scale becomes more apparent.